ALL YOU WANTED TO KNOW ABOUT
Kidney

Edited by
Dr Savitri Ramaiah

New Dawn

NEW DAWN
An imprint of Sterling Publishers (P) Ltd.
A-59 Okhla Industrial Area, Phase-II, New Delhi-110020.
Tel: 6387070, 6386209 Fax: 91-11-6383788
E-mail: ghai@nde.vsnl.net.in
www.sterlingpublishers.com

All You Wanted to Know About - Kidney Stones
© 2000, Sterling Publishers Private Limited
ISBN 81 207 2305 8

Reprint 2002, 2004

All rights are reserved. No part of this publication may be reproduced, stored in a retrieval system or transmitted, in any form or by any means, mechanical, photocopying, recording or otherwise, without prior written permission of the publisher.

Published by Sterling Publishers Pvt. Ltd., New Delhi-110016
Lasertypeset by Vikas Compographics, New Delhi-110029.
Printed at : Sai Early Learners (P) Ltd.

Information for this series, has been provided by *Health Update*, a monthly bulletin of the Society for Health Education and Learning Packages. The Update is intended to provide you with knowledge to adopt preventive measures and cooperate with the doctor during illness for better outcome of treatment.

Contributors

ALLOPATHY
Dr Sanjeev Saxena
(Consultant Nephrologist, Pushpavati Singharia Research Institute, New Delhi)

AYURVEDA
Dr V N Pandey
(Former Director, Central Council for Research in Ayurveda and Siddha, New Delhi)

HOMOEOPATHY
Dr Sangeeta Chopra
(Consultant Homoeopathy, New Delhi)

NATURE CURE
Dr Sambhashiva Rao
(Consultant, Naturopathy, Pandrapadu, Dist. Guntur, Andhra Pradesh)

UNANI
Hakim Mohammed Khalid Siddiqui
(Director, Central Council for Research in Unani, New Delhi)

Preface

All You Wanted to Know About is an easy-to-read reference series put together by *Health Update* and assisted by a team of medical experts who offer the latest perspectives on body health.

Each book in the series enhances your knowledge on a particular health issue. It makes you an active participant by giving multiple perspectives to choose from — allopathy, acupuncture, ayurveda, homoeopathy, nature cure and unani.

This book is intended as a home adviser but does not substitute a doctor.

The opinions are those of the contributors, and the publisher holds no responsibility.

Contents

Preface   4
Introduction   6
Allopathy   9
Ayurveda   73
Homoeopathy   97
Nature Cure   113
Unani   141
Definitions   148

Introduction

Kidney stones are one of the most painful conditions and have been affecting people for several centuries. They are one of the most common disorders of the urinary tract. Kidney stones are a major problem and an important cause of kidney failure in India. Appropriate and timely treatment of kidney stones can prevent severe complications such as kidney failure.

Stones in the urinary tract are a common disorder because urine is a chemical solution that contains a large number of chemical substances. These substances can crystallize easily and then grow in size to form stones.

The number of people suffering from kidney stones is increasing every year, especially in the industrially developed countries. It is relatively less common in places where the economy is based on agriculture. This highlights the role of affluence and dietary factors in formation of kidney stones.

In India, stones in the urinary tract are very common in the sub-Himalayan region from Punjab to North-East. This is why this region is known as "the stone belt".

Kidney stones are more common among men than in women.

ALLOPATHY

What are the kidneys?

The kidneys are large bean shaped organs located below the ribs on both sides of the backbone.

Each kidney is about four to five inches long and two to two and a half inches thick. It is roughly the size of your fist.

The inner side of the kidneys is concave and has a slit-like opening. The arteries, veins, nerves and the ureters are connected to the kidney through this opening into a cavity inside the kidneys.

The two main arteries of the kidneys first divide into four or five branches.

Subsequently, they divide into smaller and smaller branches, till each small branch leads to a compact ball of small blood vessels, the capillaries, called the *glomerulus*.

It allows water and wastes to pass through its walls so that they can be excreted out as urine. Glomerulus are the main filtering units of *nephrons*, which are the functional units of the kidneys.

There are more than one million nephrons in each kidneys.

About one hundred and eighty litres of blood is filtered by the kidneys everyday.

At the end of the filtration, it forms about one and a half litres of urine everyday. The remaining is absorbed back into the body through the arteries.

They filter the blood and remove excess water and wastes from it and convert it into urine. They also maintain the normal balance of various chemical substances in the blood.

The urine formed in all the functional parts of the kidney is collected in a reservoir called the *pelvis* of the kidneys. It is like a funnel.

The urine enters through its broad end and passes out of its narrow end into the *ureter*. The ureter is a fourteen to eighteen inch tube that arises from each kidney.

It transports urine from the kidney to the *urinary bladder*. The urine is stored in the bladder till it is discharged from the body. The structure of the urinary tract is as illlustrated in Figure 1.

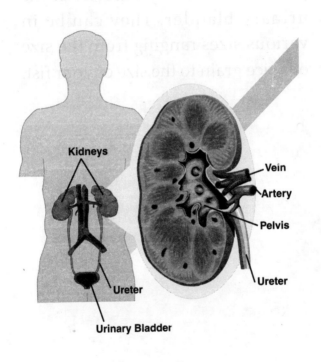

Figure 1: The urinary tract

Stones can form anywhere in the pelvis of the kidneys, ureters or the urinary bladder. They can be in various sizes ranging from the size of a rice grain to the size of your fist.

How are kidney stones formed?

As mentioned earlier, urine is a chemical solution that contains large number of substances that are dissolved in it.

Many of these chemical substances are sparingly soluble and as soon as any one of them is in excess, it forms crystals. The crystals grow over a period of time and become stones.

Chemical substances that normally form stones include

calcium, phosphate, oxalate, uric acid and cystine.

Most of these minerals are present in the urine in a concentration that is just below the level where they are soluble. This is why they normally remain as solutions and do not form crystals.

The urine of people who have kidney stones contains these minerals more frequently and has a tendency to form crystals more easily than in normal people.

It is important to remember that presence of crystals in the urine does not always lead to formation of stones in the urinary tract. Normal people tend to pass crystals of calcium phosphate, calcium oxalate and uric acid in their urine and never develop kidney stones.

This is because of two main reasons:

1. The concentration of the chemical substances is never in the range of super-saturation; and

2. The level of chemical substances that inhibit crystallization of some chemical substances in the urine is high.

3. Substances that inhibit crystallization in the urine include magnesium, citrate, pyrophosphates and several other molecules that promote minerals to remain in a soluble form.

What are the high risk groups for developing kidney stones?

Described below are the factors that increase the risk of development of kidney stones. These factors are listed in Box 1.

- Decreased concentration of chemical substances that inhibit crystallization of other chemical substances;

- Increased concentration of chemical substances that have a tendency to crystallize;

Box 1: Risk factors for development of kidney stones

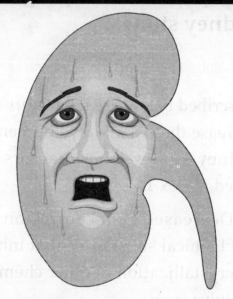

General factors

- Decreased concentration of chemical substances such as magnesium, citrate, pyrophosphates, etc. These substances inhibit formation of crystals in the urine.

- Increased concentration of chemical substances such as calcium, phosphate, oxalate, uric acid and cystine. These substances promote formation of crystals in the urine.
- Drinking less volume of fluids.
- Increased exposure to sun and excessive sweating.
- Kidney stones in other family members, especially blood relatives.
- Stress.
- Passing less than one litre of urine per day.
- Sedentary lifestyle.

- Increased intake of dairy products, animal meat and low fibre diets.

Underlying diseases

- Increased activity of the parathyroid glands. These are two pairs of endocrine glands that are situated behind the thyroid gland in the front of the neck. They produce a hormone that increases the level of calcium in the blood by mobilising it from the bones.

- Increased level of oxalic acids or oxalates in the urine. This is normally due to hereditary deficiency of an enzyme necessary to digest oxalic acid or a disorder of absorption of fat from the small intestine. Common sources of oxalic acids are fruits and vegetables.

- Disorders of the tubules in the kidneys.
- A condition in which there is abnormal presence of an amino acid called cystine in the urine. It is because of a rare inherited disease. Amino acids are chemical compounds that are building blocks of protein.
- Gout: This is a disease associated with inborn error in the utilisation of uric acid that either increases production of uric acid or interferes with its excretion of the urine.
- Any disorder that results in obstruction in the urinary tract.

- There is at least one chemical substance that can crystallize in super saturated range.
- The type of stone depends upon the chemical substance that is in excess.
- Most of the stones are calcium stones as it is the mineral most common in urine.
- Calcium can be precipitated as calcium oxalate or calcium phosphate or both.
- Uric acid is formed when protein is digested in the body and is passed out in the body.

- Excess of uric acid in the urine can lead to uric acid stones. These stones are more common among people who eat non-vegetarian foods.

- Most people who develop kidney stones tend to drink less volume of fluids.

- Drinking less fluids makes the urine very concentrated and therefore the chemical substances in it become super saturated.

- Kidney stones are also common in weather conditions that result in increased sweating.

- This is because when fluids are lost in sweat and adequate amounts are not taken orally, urine volume will be less. It will also be more concentrated.
- This is why kidney stones are more common in Gulf countries and North India.

Some other factors that increase the risk of development of kidney stones include:

- Children and siblings of people who have kidney stones are more likely to develop them as compared to those whose family members do not have them.

- It is not clear whether this is because of some hereditary factors or because of common environment factors such as diet, place of residence, etc.
- As mentioned earlier, hot weather promotes formation of stones.
- Kidney stones are more common among military personnel who are transferred from a temperate to a hot climate.
- This is because hot climate increases sweating and results in highly concentrated urine.

- Increased exposure to sunlight results in increased absorption of Vitamin D3 from the skin.

- Increased Vitamin D3 in the body leads to increased calcium absorption and therefore increased excretion in the urine.

- People with mental stress have been observed to have higher concentration of calcium, oxalate and uric acid in their urine.

- It is not clear how stress causes excessive concentration of these substances.

- People who pass less than one litre of urine per day are more likely to develop kidney stones.
- Some experts believe that drinking hard water regularly can increase the risk of kidney stones. It has, however, not yet been proven.
- Hard water contains increased amount of calcium and this is why it is believed that it can increase the risk of kidney stones.
- People who have a sedentary lifestyle or their job requires increased exposure to heat have a

higher risk of developing kidney stones.

- People who consume large portions of dairy products, refined low fibre carbohydrate diet and animal meat are at higher risk of developing kidney stones.

Sometimes kidney stones may be the result of an underlying disorder of some other organ. Some of these conditions are listed in Box 1.

What are the symptoms of kidney stones?

Many people with kidney stones do not have any symptoms. They may be detected during routine examination and tests for some other disease or problem in the abdomen.

Sometimes even very large stones, as large as the kidney itself, may also be present without causing any symptom.

- The most dramatic symptom of kidney stones is severe pain along with blood in the urine.

- The pain is in the flanks, in the left or right side depending upon the kidney in which the stone is present.

- This pain can spread down to the groin and is often associated with burning in the urine and sometimes passing gravel in the urine.

- If the stone is present in the kidney, it may just cause a dull ache or a dragging sensation in the loin.

- Stones in the ureter cause the maximum pain that often spreads to the testes or the tip of the penis in males.

- Stones may also be present in the urinary bladder although it is more commonly found in children and malnourished people.

- Bladder stones are almost never seen in developed countries.

- Stones in the urinary tract often lead to infections. This is why if you complain of frequent urinary infections, your doctor will recommend tests to detect the presence of stones, if any.

- People with repeated urinary infections are also more likely to develop kidney stones.
- These stones are normally formed of magnesium ammonium phosphate along with calcium phosphate.
- Thus, urinary infections and urinary stones form a vicious cycle.
- Repeated infections of the urinary tract can adversely affect kidney functions and even lead to kidney failure.

- Another major problem of kidney stones is obstruction to the flow of urine.
- This obstruction leads to back pressure and ballooning of the kidneys.
- Ballooning of the kidneys is called *hydronephrosis*. It is a serious complication and if not treated early, can lead to loss of kidney functions.
- Since there are two kidneys, loss of function in one kidney because of stones does not normally cause any problems.

- Often kidney stones are detected when the other kidney is also affected.
- If both the kidneys have stones, and their functions are adversely affected, it may be difficult to restore their functions to normal levels.
- Kidney stones can also cause high blood pressure. This is why it is important to conduct laboratory tests to detect the level of kidney functions in all people who have high blood pressure.

Box 2 lists the common symptoms of kidney stones.

Box 2: Symptoms of kidney stones

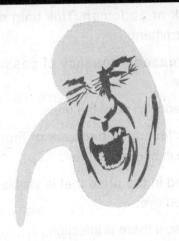

- There may be no symptoms at all.
- Severe colic like pain in the flanks that radiates to the groin, scrotum in men and labia in women.
- Nausea and vomiting.

- Dull pain that is difficult to define in the back or abdomen. This pain may be intermittent.
- Increased frequency of passing the urine.
- Urgency to pass the urine.
- Restlessness because of increased pain in some postures.
- Blood in the urine that is visible to the naked eye.
- Fever, if there is infection.

What laboratory tests are recommended for kidney stones?

There are three reasons why laboratory tests are recommended for kidney stones. These include:

- To find out the type of kidney stone;
- To identify factors contributing to the formation of kidney stones; and
- Detect damage done to the kidney by stones, if any.

Tests normally recommended for kidney stones include:

- Blood tests for urea, serum creatinine, uric acid, calcium and phosphate.
- Urine examination to detect infections, if any, and to detect the presence of crystals.
- These crystals help detect the type of stones present in the urinary tract.
- Sometimes, analysis of urine samples collected over twenty-four hours.

- This test is recommended for detecting the levels of calcium, phosphate, urate and oxalate.

- X-rays and ultrasound of the abdomen are recommended to confirm the presence of kidney stones and identify its size and location.

- Intravenous pyelography is a special x-ray test in which a contrast dye is injected into a vein.

- This contrast dye circulates to the kidneys and is excreted in the urine.

- When it collects in the ureter, it makes it opaque and therefore visible in the x-ray.
- This test thus detects obstruction in the urinary tract.

What is the treatment for kidney stones?

Detailed below are the management options for kidney stones.

Adequate water intake:

- The only convincingly proven treatment for kidney stones is to ensure adequate intake of fluids.

- It is desirable that you drink the volume of fluids enough to make you pass at least two litres of urine per day.

- This means that you must drink water both during the day and night. You will need to get up at night to both drink water and pass urine.

- Drinking hard water such as in the hills is not harmful as the benefits of increased water intake outweigh the likely adverse effects of higher calcium in the water.

- In case you are working in an environment that requires exposure to high temperatures, you are more likely to have excess sweating and dehydration. You should therefore consume more water at frequent intervals.

It is important to remember that if you are drinking adequate water, your urine will be clear, just like water. A tinge of yellow means that the urine is concentrated and you need to drink more water regularly.

Medicines:

- Your doctor may recommend some medicines that control the amount of acid or alkali in the urine because they are the key factor in formation of stones.

- A medicine called *Allopurinol* is recommended if you have high uric acid level as this medicine lowers the level of uric acid.

- There are some medicines that reduce calcium level in the blood and therefore benefit people who have kidney stones and high calcium levels.

- A medicine called *hydrochlorothiazide* decreases the amount of calcium released by the kidneys into the urine and therefore can prevent calcium stones.

- Another medicine called sodium cellulose phosphate binds calcium in the intestines and prevents it from leaking into the urine.

- A medicine called *thiola* is sometimes recommended if you have cystine stones because it reduces the amount of cystine in the urine. Medicines can prevent recurrence of kidney stones.

- In case of kidney stones because of infections, your doctor is likely to recommend antibiotics to prevent bacterial infection after the stones are removed.

- He/she will also recommend urine tests at regular intervals to detect bacteria in the urine, if any, at the earliest.

- In case the stones cannot be removed because of infections, a newer medicine called *acetohydroamic acid* may be recommended with antibiotics to prevent infections.

Surgical treatment:

- Surgery is the mainstay of treatment of kidney stones. Indications for surgery for kidney stones are as listed in Box 3.

Box 3: Indications for surgery in kidney stones

- The stone does not pass out on its own and is causing constant or severe pain.
- The stone is very large and cannot pass out of the urinary tract on its own.
- The stone blocks or obstructs the flow of urine.
- The stone leads to urinary tract infection.
- There is damage to the kidney functions.
- Blood is constantly passed out in the urine.

- In recent times there have been several newer techniques that require a smaller cut in the skin to remove the stones and therefore a shorter stay in the hospital.

Detailed below are the surgical options for treatment of kidney stones.

Percutaneous surgery:

- In this procedure, a hole is made in the skin through which instruments are passed in the body so that they reach the kidneys directly.

- Special instruments are used to either break the stone into small parts or remove it.
- A large number of kidney stones can be removed through this procedure.
- The success rate of percutaneous surgery for kidney stones is more than ninety-five per cent.
- You may have to stay in the hospital for a few days after this procedure.
- A tube may be left in the body for drainage from the site of the procedure during the recovery period.

Lithotripsy:

- A group of engineers in Germany recognised that focussed shock waves could disintegrate kidney stones. They collaborated with doctors to develop lithotripsy machine.

- In this procedure, shockwaves created outside the body are made to travel through the skin and body tissues till they hit the kidney stones.

- The impact of these shockwaves results in breaking down of the stone to smaller sand-like particles.

- There are different methods of lithotripsy. None of these methods require any cuts in the body. Most of them require anesthesia for a short time.

- Sometimes, x-rays or ultra-sound machines are also used with lithotripsy to help your doctor target the shockwaves on the stones correctly.

- During the procedure you may feel pressure on the back, as if someone is thumping it. You will, however, not feel any pain. The procedure may last up to one hour.

- Lithotripsy may lead to some minor complications. You are likely to have mild pain or discomfort in the abdomen at the place from where shockwaves had passed into the body.

- There may be blood in the urine for a few days after treatment.

- Sometimes, the smaller particles of the stones may cause pain and discomfort when they pass through the urinary tract along with the urine.

- Sometimes the stone may not break into small sand-like

particles and surgical procedures may therefore be required to remove the stone.

- Hard stones may require more than one session of lithotripsy to break the stone into small parts and sometimes they may not break at all.

Endoscopic stone surgery:

- In this procedure, your doctor will pass a flexible tube into the urinary bladder through the urethra.
- He/she will remove stones that are located either in the ureter or urinary bladder with the help of

wire baskets that catch the stones.

- This procedure is recommended for stones in the lower part of the ureter near the bladder.

Open surgery:

- About five per cent people with kidney stones are likely to require open surgery, especially if the stones are large or impacted within the kidney.

- During the surgery, the doctor will cut the skin about five to ten inches long.

- Next, he/she will cut the underlying tissues including the kidney and remove the stone manually.

- You are likely to completely recover from the surgery within four to six weeks.

What is the role of diet in kidney stones?

As mentioned earlier, it is important that you drink large volume of water, more than two litres so that you pass at least two litres of urine per day.

Water plays a very vital role in management of all types of kidney stones irrespective of their cause.

Drinking large volume of water will dilute the urine and prevent crystallization of minerals that can form the stones.

The main aim of dietary management is to correct defect in the chemical processes during digestion, absorption and utilization of the minerals.

Your doctor will recommend decrease in the intake of high risk foods and increase foods that can inhibit formation of stones.

More than seventy-five per cent of the stones are either calcium oxalate or calcium phosphate. Of these two, calcium oxalate stones are more common.

The recommended dietary allowance for calcium is four

hundred to five hundred milligrams per day. To get this amount of calcium, you need to limit milk and milk products to a maximum of one cup per day. You also need to reduce intake of calcium rich foods. These include:

- Cheese, skimmed milk, *khoya*
- Fish and sea food such as crab, *chingri*, shrimp, snail
- *Rajmah*, soyabean
- *Til* (Sesame), poppy seeds, lime peel
- *Phalsa*

- Curry leaves, black *arbi* leaves, fenugreek leaves
- Jaggery

Oxalates in the urine precipitate with calcium to form calcium oxalate stones. You should therefore avoid foods rich in oxalate. Box 4 lists the content of oxalates in various types of food.

Uric acid stones:

- These stones are associated with the disease called gout.
- Aspirin can increase the excretion of uric acid in the urine and therefore promote formation of uric acid stones.

Box 4: Oxalate content of common foods

Foods	Little oxalate	Moderate oxalate	High oxalate
Beverages	Lemonade, Red or white wine, Beer, Carbonated cola	Coffee	Tea, Cocoa
Milk	Butter milk, Yogurt, Whole and skimmed milk		
Meats	Eggs, Cheese, Poultry, Fish, Shellfish		Tofu, Baked beans
Vegetables	Cauliflower, Cabbage, Onions, Mushroom, Peas, Potatoes, Radish	Broccoli, Corn, Carrots, Lettuce, Tomato, Turnip, Arbi, Sweet Potato, Kamalkakri	Beets, Beet leaves, Beans, Brinjal, Cholai, Ladies fingers, Capsicum, Spinach

Fruits	Banana, Green grapes, Grapefruit, Mango, Melons	Apple, Apricots, Cherries, Plums, Prunes	Black grapes, Strawberries, Lime peel, Figs, Amla, Phalsa
Cereals	Macaroni, Rice, Noodles, Bread	Corn	
Fats	Vegetable Oils, Butter, Margarine		
Miscellaneous	Coconut		Peanuts, Almonds, Walnuts, Cashew nuts, Chocolates, Cocoa, Marmalade, Til Seeds, Tomato Soup

- The most important factor responsible for this type of stone formation is acidic urine.

- They are therefore treated by providing adequate fluids and by raising the normally acidic urine to a pH of 6-6.5.

- This is done by increasing the intake of alkaline foods and supplements of citrates and bicarbonates.

- If the concentration of uric acid is very high, your doctor is likely to recommend restriction of protein in the diet.

- It is also important to reduce or avoid foods rich in purine. You also need to avoid excess tea, coffee and cocoa.

Box 5 lists the purine content of common foods.

Since diet influences the acidity and alkalinity of urine, it is important to modify the diet in such a way that the pH of the urine is maintained.

- Most fruits and vegetables make the urine alkaline whereas high protein foods, bread, cereals, etc., make the urine acidic.

Box 5: Purine content in common foods

Low Purine Foods

Milk, Eggs, Cheese, All cereals except oats

Moderately Rich Purine Foods

Poultry, Fish, Peas, Lentils, Beans, Spinach, Mushrooms

High Purine Foods

Glandular meats such as liver, kidneys and brain, Sardines, Meat broth

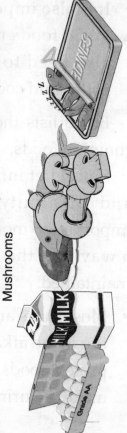

- Normally, you need to avoid excessive intake of these foods rather than avoid them completely.

Box 6 lists the acidic and alkaline foods.

It is important to remember that although the signs and symptoms of different types of kidney stones are similar, their treatment including dietary recommendations depend upon the type of stones. You should therefore strictly follow your doctor's advice, especially for the diet.

Box 6: Neutral, alkaline and acidic foods

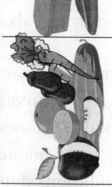

Neutral Foods

Butter, Oils, Sugar, Honey, Arrowroot, Corn, Tapioca, Coffee, Tea

Alkaline Foods

Milk and its products, Cream, Buttermilk, Almonds, Coconut, All vegetables except corn, All fruits except plums and prunes

Acidic Foods

Meat, Fish, Eggs, Cheese, Peanuts, Walnuts, Breads and other cereals, Noodles, Rice, Cakes, Pulses, Plums, Prunes

If you blindly restrict some foods that promote stone formation, it may actually harm you. You should therefore try to reduce the urinary risk factors through natural components of diet.

For example, tartaric acid in tamarind reduces urinary risk factors for formation of kidney stones.

AYURVEDA

Kidney stones are called *Ashmari* in Ayurveda. According to this system, although there have been several new surgical methods for management of kidney diseases including kidney stones, conservative management of kidney stones is still considered to be more effective.

Ashmari is described in several ancient scriptures of Ayurveda. These scriptures have recommended herbo-mineral preparations for treatment of kidney stones.

In addition to Ayurvedic medicines, several folklore medicines including tribal medicines have also been found to be effective in dissolving and/or disintegrating stones in the kidneys or urinary bladder.

Charaka, the ancient Ayurvedic physician, has emphasised the role of quality and quantity of food in various diseases.

He observed that food substances may have the right balance with the *doshas* (bio-force) but it is not necessary that they act in harmony to the mechanisms of balance that are preserved by the *dhatus* (supporting tissues of the body).

Ashmari is considered to be due to a defect in the normal functions of the urinary passages.

Ayurveda recognises that kidneys are responsible for selective absorption and excretion but it is also an important organ that deals with the flow and regulation of the digestion and utilisation of fat.

This is why kidneys are supposed to be the root of flow of

medavaha shrotas (fat tissue or substances that take part in digestion and utilization of fats).

Ayurveda has also identified kidneys to be directly involved in the other diseases such as urinary tract disorders, diabetes and obesity.

In addition to these conditions, kidney stones can also be formed because of frequent voluntary control of the urge to pass urine, reduced intake of water or having food or indulging in sex after voluntary control of the urge to pass urine.

Charaka has recommended that the principles of treatment of pain while passing urine should be applied for management of all diseases of the urinary system.

Sushruta, the famous ancient Ayurvedic surgeon has observed that kidney stones are formed due to drying of *shelashma* (mucus like material that forms the centre of the kidney stones). He described four types of kidney stones. These include:

- Kaphaashmari or phosphate stones
- Pittaashmari or uric acid stones

- Vataashmari or oxalate stones
- Shukraashmari or spermatic concretion found only in adult males and not in children.

What are the symptoms of kidney stones?

Ayurveda describes the following symptoms of kidney stones:

- Severe pain in the abdomen, in the umbilical area or lower middle area (region of the urinary bladder) that may spread to the penis or perineum.

- Obstruction to the flow of urine because of which urine is passed with difficulty. The urine may also be passed drop by drop.

- Severe pain while passing the urine.
- Severe pain in the region of the bladder that worsens by running, jumping, riding and walking long distance.
- Blood passed in the urine.

What is the treatment of kidney stones?

Ayurveda recommends a wide range of medicines for treatment of kidney stones. The choice of treatment depends upon your symptoms, severity of the disease and the type of stones.

In addition to herbal medicines, there are several folklore medicines also that have been observed to be very effective for treatment of kidney stones. It is important to remember that you should avoid taking these folklore medicines without consulting your physician as taking the wrong medicine or in the wrong dosage can worsen your condition and/or harm you.

Some of the commonly recommended medicines for kidney stones include:

- Forty to eight grams of powdered seeds of *Kulattha* (dolichos bean) to be taken twice a day.

- Four grams of the powdered fruit of *Goksura* (small caltrops) added with adequate honey to make a paste and taken twice a day.

- You should drink two hundred and fifty millilitres of cow's milk or sheep's milk after taking this medicine.
- Five grams of powdered seeds of *auruvaru* and *trapashu* to be taken with grape juice and saffron.

Some of the **folklore medicines** for kidney stones are:

Abutilon asiaticum *G. Don (H. Kanghi).*
- This is an undershrub with yellow flowers and is available in Bundelkhand, Central and South India.

- The leaves are applied internally for stones in the urinary bladder.

Centtaurea calcitrappa *Linn.*

- This is a rigid herb with purple flowers and grows in North-Western India, in Punjab, Kashmir and in Mysore.

- The root is considered as a cure for gravel and its powdered seeds are taken with wine for kidney stones. This tree grows up to a height of over one thousand metres.

Dichrostachys cinera *W and A (S. Viravriksha, H. Vurtuli).*

- This is a shrub with minute flowers, the upper part of which is fertile and lower sterile.

- It has purple or rose coloured stamen nodes and grows in the Upper Gangetic Plains, Central and South India.

- The root is used to break the large stones into smaller pieces in the urinary tract.

Homonoia riparia *Lour (S. Pashanbhedaka, Kumaon, Kandagar).*

- This is a rigid evergreen willow-like shrub that grows in Bengal,

Assam, Khasi Hills, Bundelkhand, Central and Western India and the Andaman Islands.

- The decoction of the root is recommended for discharges from the urinary tract and stones in the urinary bladder.

Prunnus cerasoides *D. Don syn. P. puddum Roxb. ex Wall (S. Padmaka, H and Kumaon, Paddam).*

- This is a large tree with brilliant flowers that are red or white in colour.
- It grows in temperate Himalayas in Garhwal at the height of nine

hundred to eighteen hundred metres and in Sikkim and Bhutan at a height of fifteen hundred to twenty-four hundred metres.

- The kernel is used to treat gravel and kidney stones.

Simple medicines recommended for treatment of kidney stones include:

- Fourteen to twenty-eight millilitres of decoction prepared from twelve grams bark of *Varuna*, two grams of dried ginger and six grams of the fruit of small caltrops.

- This medicine is recommended with half a gram of *Yavakshara* and twenty-five grams of jaggery twice a day.

- Fourteen to twenty-eight millilitres of decoction prepared from equal parts of *Varuna*, rhizome of saxifrage, dried ginger and fruit of small caltrops is recommended with half a gram of *Yavakshara* twice a day.

- Fourteen to twenty-eight millilitres of decoction prepared from equal parts of cardamom, roots of long pepper and *Madhuyasti* (glycyrrhiza), bark of horseradish, leaf of *vasaka*, rhizome of saxifrage, seed of *Renuka*, fruit of small caltrops and root and bark of castor.

- This decoction is recommended with five grams of *shuddha silajatu*, twenty-five grams of raw sugar and fourteen grams of honey twice a day.

- Fourteen to twenty-eight millilitres of decoction prepared from equal parts of roots of sacred grass (*kusa*), sugarcane, *Kasa*, *Sara* and *Darbha*, seed of dolichos bean, bark of *Varuna* and fruit of small caltrops is recommended with twenty-five grams of raw sugar and half a gram of *Yavakshara* twice a day.

- Fourteen to twenty-eight millilitres of decoction prepared from equal parts of fruit of small caltrops, dried ginger, leaf of castor and bark of *Varuna* is recommended twice a day.

Compound preparations recommended for treatment of kidney stones include:

- Fourteen to twenty-eight millilitres of *Brhat Varunaid Kvathga* to be taken with half a gram of *Yavakshara* twice a day.

- One to two pills of *Chandraprabha vati, Gosuradi Guggulu, Pashanavajrak Rasa* and *Trivikrama Rasa* to be taken with water twice a day.

What are the dietary recommendations for kidney stones?

Ayurveda recommends old Sali variety of rice, seeds of dolichos bean, ginger, fruit of Kumanda and leaves of Salparni and Varuna for kidney stones.

What are the conditions that aggravate kidney stones?

Three types of foods can aggravate kidney stones:

- Foods that are incompatible to you;
- Acidic foods;
- Inadequate fibre or foods that cause constipation.

Suppression of the natural urge to pass urine can also aggravate or cause kidney stones.

HOMOEOPATHY

The signs, symptoms of kidney stones and its types in the Homoeopathic system of medicine are the same as those detailed in the section on Allopathy. Practitioners of Homoeopathy opine that most kidney stones and the symptoms they cause can be cured with medicines. They are especially effective for those who are not able to undergo surgical procedure or who have repeated episodes of kidney stones.

How do Homoeopathic medicines act on kidney stones?

There are three main ways in which Homoeopathic medicines act on kidney stones. These include:

- Dissolving the large stones into granules
- Improving the kidney functions by increasing their excretory functions
- Mobilising the gravel of the kidney stones to move into the

ureter and then pass out with the urine.

In addition to the above, Homoeopathic medicines are also effective in controlling infections and reducing the risk of formation of kidney stones again. Homoeopathic practitioners opine that these medicines are especially effective for those who have a tendency for recurrent kidney stones.

What is the Homoeopathic approach for treatment of kidney stones?

Just as for all diseases, Homoeopathy lays special emphasis on taking the history of your symptoms. Your doctor will ask detailed questions about the following:

- History of similar complaints in other family members
- Your habits, likes, dislikes, mental attitude, etc.

- Exact location of pain, including the site of origin and its spread
- The side where the pain is more (left or right)
- Type of pain, such as pricking, burning, etc.
- Factors that aggravate or relieve the symptoms
- Colour, frequency, quantity and smell of the urine.

What is the treatment for kidney stones?

Detailed below are the Homoeopathic medicines commonly recommended for treatment of kidney stones.

Berberis vulgaris:

This is the most frequently used medicine for treatment of kidney stones. Although it is normally recommended as the medicine of choice for kidney stones, it is especially effective in the following situations: stone in the left kidney with tearing or cutting type of pain extending from the loin to the groin.

The urine is hot, burning with blood and grey or red sediments. This medicine dissolves the stones and expels them along with urine. It is normally recommended as tincture.

Lycopodium:

- This medicine is effective for stones in the right side of the kidney with red sediments in the urine, severe backache that is relieved by passing urine, pain that is worse in the evening and associated indigestion and increased gas in the bowels.

- It is also recommended for people who are short-tempered, have a dominating personality and a marked craving for sweets and hot drinks.

Ocimum Can:

- It is recommended for stones in the right kidney with red sand in the urine.
- It is very effective for uric acid stones, muddy urine with musk-like smell.

Sepia:

- This medicine is normally recommended for reddish sediments in urine associated with involuntary urination in the sleep.
- It is especially effective for those who complain of bearing down sensation in the pelvis and women who have menstrual irregularities.
- Most people with these symptoms are likely to be depressed, irritable and indifferent to family issues.

Benzoic Acid:

- This medicine is recommended for offensive and ammonia-like smell of the urine. It is also effective for uric acid stones that result in sharp shifting pain and associated gout.

Cantharis:

- It is recommended for severe cutting and burning type of pain in the back, in the area where the kidneys are located.

- It is also recommended for painful and scanty urine with constant urge to pass urine. It is also effective in urinary tract infections in people with kidney stones.

Sarsaparilla:

- This medicine is recommended for colic-like pain and pain while passing urine, especially in children. These children scream and cry before and while passing the urine. An important symptom is pain at the end of passing the urine.

Magnesia Phos and Colocynth:

- These two medicines are very effective for colic-like pain and act as efficient analgesics.

- Magnesia Phos is especially effective for cramp-like pain that worsens with cold temperature and touch and reduces by warmth and bending forwards.
- Colocynth is effective for intense burning pain in the abdomen while passing urine and the pain reduces with hard pressure.

Nitric acid:

- This medicine is normally recommended for calcium oxalate crystals in urine that smells like horse's urine and is associated with burning type of pain and passing albumin in the urine.

The above medicines are deep acting and have wide range of effects. Your doctor is the best person to decide on the medicine and its dose that is most suited to you.

In addition to the above, Homoeopathy also recommends increased intake of fluids, moderate diet, avoiding red meat and a diet that is rich in calcium, cholesterol and uric acid.

Limitations of Homoeopathy for this treatment.

Homoeopathic medicines are not effective for the following conditions.

- Large stones that are more than three centimetres in size
- Stones in the lower part of the kidney
- Acute obstruction in the kidneys or ureter
- Distension and dilatation of the pelvis of the kidney due to obstruction.

NATURE CURE

The signs, symptoms and type of kidney stones as per Nature Cure are the same as those detailed in the section on Allopathy. According to this system of medicine, when the process of elimination of toxins from the kidney is adversely affected the level of toxins in the body increases. These toxins can deposit in the urinary system, either in the kidneys, ureters, bladder or urethra.

These deposits gradually increase in size, form stones and finally interfere with the kidney function and/or passage of urine.

Nature Cure also recommends ultrasound tests and x-rays to determine the existence of kidney stones, their size, number and exact location. Depending upon the findings of these tests, several physical measures and dietary modifications are recommended for management of kidney stones.

What is the treatment for kidney stones?

The treatment of kidney stones depends upon their size and location. Sometimes the symptoms may be mild and natural methods can then be adopted to treat the stones and prevent their recurrence. In case the symptoms are very severe, surgical treatment is often necessary.

The main aim of treatment for kidney stones as per Nature Cure is to remove toxins from the body as soon as they are formed.

Since kidneys are one of the main routes of removing toxins, they are stimulated with appropriate treatment measures.

Other treatment measures include alkaline diet rich in minerals and neutralisation of toxins formed at the end of digestion immediately.

Nature Cure recommends the following measures for management of kidney stones:

Drinking water:

- Nature Cure recommends drinking large volume of water as the first step towards dissolving kidney stones, facilitating their passage in the urine and preventing recurrence of kidney stones.

- About two to two and a half litres of water is recommended per day.

- Some Nature Cure practitioners recommend about six to eight litres a day for those who have kidney stones.

- Water dilutes the concentration of fluids in various parts of the body and makes it easier for the kidneys to filter blood.

- It is important that you drink water at frequent intervals so that the total volume of fluid is maintained in the body and the concentration of toxins in all body parts and fluids is less.

- Drinking one or two large glasses of water before going to bed at night and two to three glasses of water as soon as you wake up can prevent kidney stones.

- Drinking water just before going to bed at night helps neutralise toxins that are formed at night.

- Many people tend to ignore the urge to pass urine or drink less water so that they do not have the urge to pass urine very frequently.

- This is not desirable. This is because if the urine is not passed, the concentration of toxins in the urine will increase.

- When the toxins increase, the salt content in them is deposited in the urinary system. Over a period of time, they form kidney stones.

Hot hip bath:

- A hot hip bath is recommended if you have pain because of kidney stones. Taking a hip bath involves sitting in a hip bath tub filled with hot water at a temperature you can tolerate just for ten to fifteen minutes.

- It should be immediately followed by a cold shower for two minutes.

Alternate hot and cold water:

- Pain due to kidney stones can also be relieved by sitting alternately in a hot water tub for three minutes and half a minute in a cold water tub.

- You need to repeat this process four to five times ending with a cold hip bath.

- You can take alternate hot and cold water bath everyday for three days and later twice a week till the stones are passed out in the urine.

Cold hip bath:

- Cold hip bath improves kidney functions and acts as a tonic for the urinary system.

- It also reduces inflammation of the kidneys and ureters.
- You can take cold hip bath for twenty minutes everyday.

Fomentation:

- You can also foment the middle back with a hot water bottle for six to ten minutes.
- Keep the middle of the back covered with a wet cloth.

Bath tub:

- In case you do not have access to hip bath tub, you can recline in a bath tub filled with hot water for fifteen minutes.

Hot pack:

- In case you do not have access to a bath tub also, you can dip a towel in hot water.
- Squeeze it slightly to remove excess water and wrap it around the abdomen for twenty minutes.
- During this time, you need to dip the towel in hot water every time the towel becomes cold.

Alternate hot and cold towel:

- Applying towel dipped in hot and cold water alternately to the middle of the back for three and one and a half minutes.

- This can also relieve pain due to kidney stones.

Kidney douche:

- This involves application of cold water for ten to fifteen minutes with a little pressure on the lower one-third of the breast bone.

- Kidney douche helps contraction of blood vessels of the kidneys and therefore increases the pressure of filtration of blood by the kidneys.

- Increased pressure while filtration will in turn increase the volume of urine produced.

Hot and cold douche:

- Applying hot and cold douche alternately can also relieve pain due to kidney stones.

Hot blanket pack:

- Cover the body with wet cloth and also with blanket.
- This results in sweating and removal of toxins from the body.
- Hot blanket pack can prevent recurrence of kidney stones.

Massage:

- A light massage to the middle back and lower back before a hot water bath can relieve pain and help remove small kidney stones.

Enema:

- A hot water enema can also stimulate kidneys and improve their functions.

All the above measures relieve pain due to kidney stones, keep urinary system active, remove toxins from the body without any delay and strengthen the urinary tract.

What are the dietary recommendations for kidney stones?

According to Nature Cure, if appropriate diet is not taken, other measures to control and prevent kidney stones will not be effective in the long run.

The main aim of diet therapy is to take large volume of alkaline minerals and reduce the amount of toxins produced as a result of digestion.

This can be achieved with natural, simple, unprocessed and wholesome foods. Salads, fruits, steamed vegetables and green leafy vegetables are most suited for people with kidney stones.

Other dietary measures recommended for kidney stones include:

Reduced intake of calcium and protein.
- Nature Cure opines that calcium derived from the organic foods is utilised by the body and therefore can be taken.

- However, calcium derived from inorganic forms such as in calcium supplements, tobacco, pan, etc., is not utilised by the body and should therefore be avoided.
- When the body does not utilise calcium, they tend to deposit in the kidneys and over a period of time form stones.
- It is desirable that you limit the intake of legumes and avoid animal protein such as dairy products, meat, etc.
- Increased intake of proteins increases the risk of some types

of kidney stones, especially uric acid stones.

Increased intake of positive alkaline minerals:

- The kidneys and skin remove toxins in the form of neutralised salts.

- This means that the salts are produced when the alkaline minerals combine with toxins that are acidic in nature.

- The toxins produced by the body combine with alkaline minerals such as iron, calcium, sodium, potassium, magnesium and manganese to form salts.

- These salts need to be removed from the body immediately as otherwise they tend to deposit in the kidneys.
- If you consume large volumes of foods rich in alkaline minerals, they will combine with toxins and enable them to be excreted from the body.

Reduce salt intake:

- Excessive use of salt increases the burden on the kidneys and therefore adversely affects its function. Poor kidney functions can lead to kidney stones.

Reduce carbohydrate intake:

- Excessive intake of carbohydrate leads to increased volume of waste products.
- It is desirable that you eat meals that contain sixty to eighty percent of total volume as vegetables and fruits and forty to twenty percent carbohydrates and proteins in the form of legumes.

Fasting:

- Nature Cure recommends fasting only after eating a neutral diet for at least two weeks in order to neutralise and remove the toxins.

Avoid spices:

- It is desirable that you avoid all stimulants, spices and beverages such as tea and coffee.

- Many people believe that people who have kidney stones should not consume tomatoes and spinach as they contain oxalic acid.

- Nature Cure does not agree with this belief. According to Nature Cure, you can take these vegetables in their natural form and in combination with other vegetables and fruits.

Kidney beans:

- Some practitioners of Nature Cure have observed that kidney beans can effectively control kidney stones.

- To prepare the medicine, you need to remove the beans inside the pods and then slice the pods.

- Put about sixty milligrams of the pods in four litres of hot water and boil it at low flame for about four hours.

- Strain the boiled liquid and allow it to cool.
- While it is cooling, do not disturb or mix the liquid.
- After about seven to eight hours, strain it again without stirring.
- You need to drink this decoction every two hours for the first two days and then several times a week.
- Avoid drinking liquid that is more than a day old as it may not be effective.

Herbal remedies:

Nature Cure recommends the following herbal remedies for treatment of kidney stones:

- *Goose berry and rose tea* as they help dissolve kidney stones.

- *Plantain tea and whey concentrate* as they help remove toxins from the body.

- *Using chopped parsley* in soups, stews, salads and spreads in their raw state improves the elimination power of the kidneys.

- *Juniper berry tea* prepared by softening six juniper berries and boiled in a cup of water improves kidney functions.

- ***Use of natural diuretics*** such as asparagus, tender coconut water, dry coriander decoction and barley water increase the volume of urine and therefore help remove toxins from the body.

- ***Use of tulsi*** juice mixed with honey several months facilitates removal of small kidney stones.

In addition to the above measures, Nature Cure also recommends regular exercises such as brisk walking, jogging and some specific exercises of yoga for improving kidney functions.

It is important that you learn the correct method of these yoga exercises before practising them everyday.

UNANI

UNANI

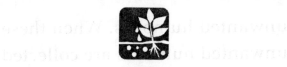

Kidney stones are known as *Hesatul Kulia* in the Unani system of medicine. According to this system, the stones are formed in the kidneys due to collection of *Ghaliz Ratubat* (thick and sticky humours) in the pelvis of the kidneys that are rich in *Arzi* particles. The body heat evaporates the *Latif* part and the *Arzi* particles settle to form base of the stones. Sometimes the body produces unwanted humours. When these unwanted humours are collected over a long period, they become thick and form the base of the kidney stones. This base of the stone is actually the centre of the kidney stones around which salts of the humours deposit to form larger stones. As the amount of salt deposits increase, the size of the stones also increase. Kidney stones may either be hard or soft.

What are the causes of kidney stones?

There are three main causes of kidney stones. These include:
- Excessive and continuous use of cold and moist food;
- Excessive use of phlegm producing diet; and
- Low water intake or drinking contaminated water.

What are the signs and symptoms of kidney stones?

The Unani system of medicine also opines that kidney stones may not result in any symptoms for a long time. They cause symptoms either when they change their position or pass down the urethra to the urinary bladder. As the stones move down to the urinary bladder, they result in severe pain. Other symptoms include burning sensation while passing the urine, blood in the urine, heaviness in the flanks and vomiting.

What is the treatment for kidney stones?

Unani system of medicine recommends single and compound medicines that break kidney stones into smaller pieces, which are then passed out in the urine.

Single medicines include Hajrul Yahood, Sang Sar-e-Mahi, Hab-ul-Qilt, Dooqoo, Kaknaj, Aaloo Baloo, Gul Tesu and Roghan Aqrab.

Compound medicines include Majoon Aqrab, Majoon Hajrul Yahood, Jawarish Zarooni and Sharbat Bazoori.

Definitions

Anus is the outer opening of the intestine from which the stools are passed out.

Arteries are large blood vessels that carry pure blood from the heart to other parts of the body.

Bladder is a bag-like structure that holds secretions. Urinary bladder holds urine.

Inflammation is a protective response of the body tissues to irritation or injury. Common signs are redness, heat, swelling and pain.

Nephrons are structural and functional units of the kidneys. They filter blood and remove waste products.

Pelvis is any structure shaped like a basin. In the human body, the term pelvis is used for the bony cage formed by the hip bones and last part of the backbone and the expanded first part of the ureter that receives urine from all filtering units of the kidneys.

Penis is the male organ that carries the urethra through which the urine and semen are discharged.

Perineum is the region of the body between the anus and the opening of the urethra. It includes both the skin and the underlying muscle. In females it is perforated by the vaginal opening.

Rectum is a portion of the large intestine just before the outer opening called the anus. It is about twelve centimetres long.

Renal is a medical term used for kidneys.

Testes are male sex organs that produce semen.

Ureters are one pair of tubes, about thirty centimetres long. They carry urine from the kidneys to the bladder.

Urethra is a small tube that drains urine from the bladder. It is short in females and long in males.

Veins are blood vessels that carry impure blood from various parts of the body to the heart.

HEALTH UPDATE

YOUR PERSONAL MEDICAL ADVISOR

SOLUTIONS FOR ANY MEDICAL PROBLEM, AT YOUR FINGERTIPS

HEALTH UPDATE gives you detailed information on common diseases and ailments from five different perspectives- **Allopathy, Ayurveda, Nature Cure, Homoeopathy** and **Unani** in a concise and easy to understand format, complete with graphic descriptions, general information, health tips and much more.

SUBSCRIPTION

India ☐ 1 year-Rs. 300/- ☐ 2 years-Rs. 500/- ☐ 3 years-Rs. 750/-
International ☐ 1 year-$25 ☐ 2 years-$45 ☐ 3 years-$60

☐ Yes, I would like to subscribe to **Health Update**, the monthly health bulletin

Name: Mr./Ms. ....
Address (mention nearest landmark)..................
....
City:.................... State:.................... Country:....................
Pin:................Tel:................Fax:................email:................
Age/Profession..................

☐ I am sending by Cheque/DD No..................drawn on (specify bank)..................for Rs..................dated..................favouring **HEALTH UPDATE**.

☐ Please charge my American Express Credit Card

Credit Card No. ☐☐☐☐☐☐☐☐☐☐☐☐☐☐☐☐☐☐☐☐☐☐☐☐☐

Card Expiry Date..................Card Holder's Signature..................

Date of Birth..................Tel. (O) ....(R)..................

Direct this subscription form to:
HEALTH UPDATE, D-31, Defence Colony, New Delhi-110024, India.
Tel.: 4622863. Fax: 91-011-4698150. email: savitri_ramaiah@vsnl.com